HEALTH
ON THE
JOB

Boost Your Immune System To Stay Healthy At Work

By Dr. Kathryn A. Boling MD

I hope that reading this book will provide you with solid strategies to improve your health, boost your immune system, and enhance your quality of life as you put in the time and the effort to excel at your job and in your career.

For more information please subscribe to my YouTube channel *Ask Dr Boling* at https://bit.ly/askdrboling

Published by Dr. Kathryn A. Boling, Baltimore MD

Printed in the United States of America.

ISBN-13: 978-1-63795-851-3

Additional copies are available at special quantity discounts for bulk purchases for sales promotions, premiums, fundraising, and educational use.

For more information, please contact: Dr. Kathryn A. Boling, DrKathrynBoling@gmail.com

Table of Contents

Healthy On The Job

When Virginia came back to work after the weekend, she was feeling tired. Initially she chalked it up to caring for her kids over the weekend. Both had become ill with mild fever and coughs Friday morning. By Monday, however, they were much improved. Their fever had resolved and their coughs were better. Virginia thought it was safe to leave them with the sitter.

In the break room she poured herself a cup of coffee and got one as well for her friend Marie, who had not yet arrived. It wasn't until just before lunch that she started to feel bad herself. Thinking that maybe she just needed to eat something, she joined a group of friends for lunch. The feeling didn't pass and by mid-afternoon she was feeling feverish and coughing in the copy room. Within two days over 20 people working on her floor were ill. The culprit: a virus. Respiratory virus can travel in the air with coughing and sneezing and then settle anywhere within a 6-foot radius. Even more worrisome, some viruses are airborne and can float around for hours, potentially infecting anyone who travels through the area.

The people who ate lunch with Virginia and mingled at work, including her boss, her friend Marie and several other office workers all unknowingly breathed in and swallowed thousands of virus particles. All of them became ill within days. Although janitorial services cleaned nightly, movement throughout the building of people newly ill caused employees in the surrounding offices to drop like dominos over the next several weeks. They became infected when they unwittingly touched doorknobs, tables and copy machine equipment that appeared clean but was in fact covered with virus particles.

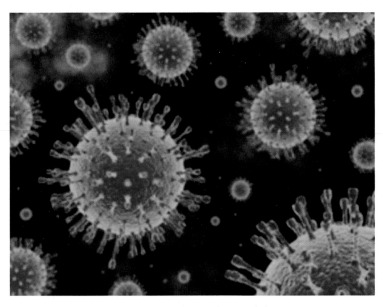

Microscopic airborne virus particles

In all, over 50 people became ill and costs to the company were significant. The story above is a fictionalized version of what is happening all over the world. But it did not start in 2019.

A 2016 study by Johns Hopkins School of Public Health estimated that one common gastrointestinal virus, norovirus, costs over 60 billion dollars globally in societal costs, with over 90% of that burden due to lost productivity. Prior to coronavirus, norovirus was the illness frequently in the news. Stories peppered the internet of cruises cancelled, cruise ships quarantined, and restaurants closed due to this common virus. Now with Covid-19, cruses are again implicated. Jails, hospitals and nursing homes have become hotspots. Air travel is decimated and multiple statewide precautions have been announced to combat this virus. But this is not a one and done situation. Unfortunately, viruses new and old are here to stay.

But what can we do? How can we keep ourselves and our families safe? Since many of us spend upwards of 40 hours on the job, strategies to keep employees healthy can do much to limit illness both on the job and at home. That is why I have written this book. I want to provide concrete information and simple strategies to help avoid illness as well as maintain the best possible health at work and at home – even if your job requires long hours and a hectic schedule.

Decrease The Risk Of Viral Illness In The Workplace

Hand washing in general reduces the risk of virus transmission. Washing your hands after using the restroom or the office kitchen can reduce the overall incidence of respiratory and gastrointestinal viral illnesses in the office.

Depending on the virus, people who are ill can be highly contagious and shed, in some cases, billions of tiny viral particles. Gastrointestinal viruses are spread in stool and vomit. Respiratory viruses spread through coughing, sneezing and sometimes even just breathing. The reason these viruses are so devastating to a business is that it takes only a few viral particles to make another person sick. Sick employees are not only contagious while they are symptomatic, but can also infect co-workers before symptoms start and possibly even after they feel better. Worst of all, symptoms can arise so suddenly that people may come to work feeling fine but become ill over the course of the workday.

With norovirus, if someone throws up in the office, the area must be immediately cleaned and disinfected to prevent an outbreak. Both contaminated surfaces and the surrounding area up to a 25-foot radius must be cleaned using a bleach-based cleaner. Persons cleaning the area should wear gloves and cover their shoes with disposable paper booties. Cleaners and anyone who was in the immediate area should wash their hands and change out of any clothes that could have come into contact with the virus.

But what about less obvious viruses, like the flu or Covid-19? Careful cleaning and limiting contact with people who are ill can help. People who are ill should be encouraged to stay home. Wearing a mask can also prevent exhaled droplets infected with virus from contaminating common areas. Wearing a mask prevents you from transmitting virus, but it does not necessarily protect you. Unless your mask is a professionally fitted N95, you are not completely protected from inhaled viral particles. That is why wearing masks AND social distancing as much as possible is necessary to prevent viral transmission. We may decide after the Covid-19 crisis is over to never go back to some of our previous behaviors, like shaking hands as a method of greeting.

Are there other things we can do to stay healthy? The answer is yes.

Healthy On The Job

Boost Your Immune System

To reduce the risk of viral and bacterial illnesses, boosting the immune system may be the most effective means of staying healthy. A strong immune system can help prevent illness as well as speed recovery should you become ill. The following factors have been shown to improve immune function:

- Stress reduction: Relaxation and/or meditation.

- A healthy diet with several servings of fruits and vegetables as well as an adequate dietary intake of Omega 3 fatty acids. Omega-3 fatty acids can reduce inflammation. Some studies have also shown it to be beneficial in boosting immune response. Multivitamins may also boost the immune system.

- Adequate sleep: Getting enough sleep is important in maintaining a healthy immune system - at least 6-7 hours a night is needed for the immune system to function adequately.

- Nurture relationships: A supportive social network (friends, a loving marital partner, relationships with extended family) can boost the immune system. Several studies have compared socially isolated people with those who have a supportive social network. People who are isolated heal slower, catch more colds, and get sick more often than those who have a supportive network. Even if we work or live alone, keeping in touch with others can help us stay healthy.

- Prevention: Get vaccinated for preventable diseases (like the flu) and get age-related medical screenings.

- Maintain a healthy-body weight with diet and regular exercise: Evidence shows that obesity and malnutrition have a negative impact on the immune system.

- Stop unhealthy behaviors: Do not smoke. If you drink alcohol, drink in moderation (no more than one alcoholic drink per day).

- Hygiene: Wash hands or sanitize frequently while at work, out in public or in any crowded place, especially during the cold and flu season. Many viruses are not only spread from infected persons coughing and sneezing around you, but are also spread object to hand and then hand to eyes or mouth after touching doorknobs or utensils. Be mindful if you are ill. Turn your head and cover your mouth with your arm when coughing (even soft coughs can spread virus droplets). Try not to cough or sneeze over food that others will eat. Remember, what appears to be a slight cold for one person could become pneumonia and an ICU admission for someone else.

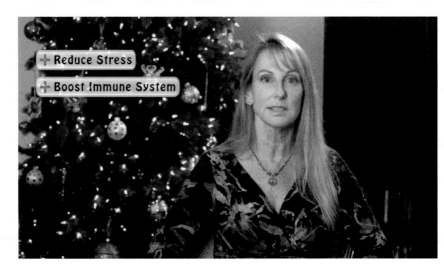

Factors That Impair Your Immune System

- Stress: Unfortunately, this is a constant for many people. Persistent high stress levels cause increased secretion of cortisol and, over time, this depresses the immune system. Stress reduction strategies described in this book can help decrease the negative effects of stress.

- Poor diet: A diet high in processed sugars can depress the immune system by impairing the body's ability to mount a defense against bacteria and viruses. Eating right and maintaining a healthy body weight can help keep the immune system healthy. Look at the labels of the foods you are eating. Becoming aware of the sugar content of what you eat can help you make healthier choices. Know that not all foods that claim to be healthy actually are.

- Depression: Untreated depression can harm the immune system. People with depression may have increased levels of cortisol, adrenaline and other stress hormones as well as increased inflammation throughout the body. This impairs the body's ability to fight off disease. Treating depression can rebalance the immune system and restore it to a healthier level. Some antidepressants boost natural killer cell activity, a potent cell that defends against viral infections and cancer. If you have noticed a persistent sad or bad mood that does not resolve in a few weeks, discuss with your doctor.

- Social disconnection can hurt the immune system. Researchers in Ohio found that people who were lonely showed signs of an impaired immune system. It turns out that they had a higher incidence of cold sores and that they produced more inflammation-related proteins than less lonely people.

- Excessive intake of alcohol also damages the immune system. While some studies show that moderate drinking may benefit the immune system (defined as seven drinks a week, no more than three drinks in any one day), heavier drinking will wreak havoc on the immune system.

- Lack of sleep has also been shown to damage the immune system. Less than 6-7 hours a night has been shown to impair the body's ability to mount an immune response to vaccines. Conversely, sleeping too much, more then 9-10 hours can also negatively impact the immune system

- Smoking cigarettes damages the immune system in many ways. There are over 7000 chemicals released when a cigarette burns. Many of them are known to cause cancer. Smoking not only causes cell damage and cancer, but it depresses immune system functions that could save your life. Damage from smoking causes a chronic level of stress as the body tries to fight off the harmful effects of continued smoking. Other chemicals, like tar, suppress the immune system further. Fortunately, once you quit smoking, over time your immune system can recover.

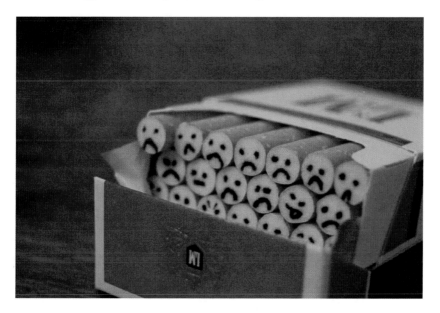

Healthy On The Job

Strategies To Keep Your Immune System Healthy: Daily Vitamin Supplements

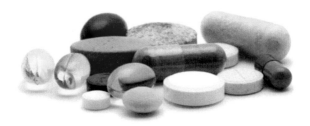

Even when you eat healthy every day (which, if you are like me and all my patients…you don't), it is hard to absorb all the necessary nutrients to keep vitamin levels sufficient to boost your immune system. To that end, I recommend the following daily vitamins:

- *Vitamin B12 1000mcg*: Vitamin B12 is good for your memory, can enhance your mood, give you energy and help with concentration and focus. It also strengthens your immune system. It can be taken either as a daily supplement or in a monthly injection for more immediate benefit. Taking this supplement in a sublingual form (dissolves under the tongue) increases oral absorption especially for persons on medications that decrease stomach acid. B12 is found primarily in red meat, so if you do not eat much red meat you should supplement with B12. Also, as we age and our immune system becomes less robust, B12 absorption also decreases, making the supplement even more important.

- *Vitamin D 2000IU-5,000IU*: Vitamin D has many important functions including improving immune system function. People with normal vitamin D levels are less likely to get the flu and, it turns out, Covid. More importantly in the long run, a normal Vitamin D level decreases the risk of heart disease and some cancers, including colon cancer. The farther north you reside or work, the more vitamin D you need to take (as your sun is further from the equator). In Baltimore I recommend my patients take 2000IU daily to maintain a low normal level of Vitamin D. If you have a cold or Covid, temporarily increasing Vitamin D intake may help you recover faster.

- *Vitamin C 500-1000mg*: Taking vitamin C regularly can reduce the incidence and duration of colds.

- *Multivitamin with minerals*: If you are like everyone else, you do not always eat a completely balanced diet. Taking a

Healthy On The Job

multivitamin can compensate for small deficits in your diet and boost your immune system in this manner.

- *Probiotic*: A recent New Zealand study showed that people taking a daily probiotic had 40% fewer colds and fewer gastrointestinal illnesses (like the Norovirus above). Try a product that does not need refrigeration.

- *Omega 3 Fish Oil*: This is a powerful anti-inflammatory supplement. Take 2000mg daily. This can help with chronic inflammation (like arthritis) and ultimately lowers cortisol levels (the stress hormone). If the Omega 3 has a disagreeable fishy aftertaste, you can freeze the vitamin before consumption.

- *Magnesium 250-500mg*: Magnesium supplementation can improve sleep, help prevent leg cramps (especially nighttime foot and calf cramping), reduce constipation and relax the nervous system. I suggest taking it at night.

- *Co-enzyme Q10 200mg*: If you suffer from heart disease, have high blood pressure or take a Statin medication to lower cholesterol you may benefit from taking this supplement. It may also help with Tinnitus (a constant or intermittent ringing or buzzing in the ear).

- *Melatonin*: 3-6 mg nightly taken 30 minutes prior to sleep can help the quality and quantity of sleep. There is anecdotal evidence that it may help with Covid recovery

- *Quercetin*: 500-1000mg daily. I have recommended this to my patients who remain symptomatic weeks after a Covid diagnosis. They have reported to me that this has helped them get better faster.

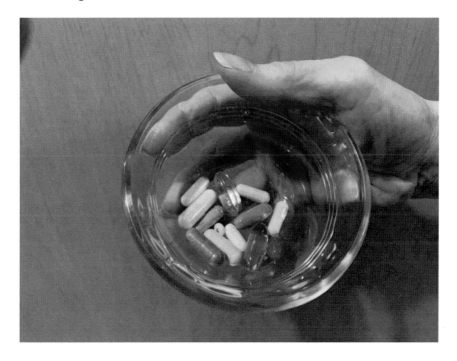

My Vitamins

Supplements To Prevent The Common Cold

Colds cause a significant amount of discomfort including nasal discharge, sore throat, sinus stuffiness and cough. Unfortunately, there is no magic pill to cure the cold, but there are some herbal supplements that, when taken as recommended, reduce your risk of catching a cold or may shorten the duration of a cold.

- *Astragalus 250-500mg (or as a tea) daily during cold and flu season (October through March):* A review from the Natural Medicine Comprehensive Database (NMCD) concluded there is evidence that taking astragalus long-term might help prevent colds. It may also be effective during allergy season to relieve symptoms of runny nose, itching and sneezing

- *Zink lozenges, pills or syrup:* Studies show taking zinc reduces the average length of a cold in healthy people. Start zinc supplementation at the first sign of a cold as it works best if taken in the first 24 hours. Zinc may also prevent the common cold as well. I take zinc 50mg, Echinacea 75mg and vitamin C 500 mg - all throughout the cold and flu season (October to April) an have continued this year into the summer due to Covid-19. I used to have a rule of 100 –

meaning I would see about 100 people with a cold and then I would get one. That gave me about 4-5 colds a year over a period of 20+ years. Then I started taking the zinc, vitamin C and Echinacea. Since then, I have had only one mild cold in 3 years. I make my husband and my medical assistant take it too (it took some convincing but they are willing now that they have seen the benefit). Pretty much on a daily basis I have people coughing literally in my face, so I believe it does prevent colds. This is backed up by a Japanese study that showed zinc taken for five months reduced the incidence of colds in children. Airborne and Zycam also contain zinc.

***Never use any nasal spray with zinc, as it can permanently impair your sense of smell.

- *Echinacea*: This herb increases the number of white blood cells, which fight infections. It has been shown to prevent cold, but used alone its effect is small. Take 500mg three times daily if you have a cold, 75 - 300mg daily to prevent colds during the cold and flu season. Do not take Echinacea if you have asthma unless you have cleared it with your doctor as it could cause asthma symptoms to worsen.

Cold And Flu Prevention And Treatment

Each year, about 20% of the US population will get the flu. Two hundred thousand of them will be hospitalized due to the severity of their illness and 3,000 – 49,000 people will die from flu complications. Now we have other viruses more deadly than the flu. With so many people working so closely together in an office environment, prevention of the flu and other viruses before they strike – and early treatment and isolation when they do – becomes paramount. The following strategies will lessen the impact from flu and other viral illnesses:

- Get a yearly flu vaccine and any other vaccines that can prevent novel viral infections (especially if you have asthma, are a smoker or have any chronic respiratory illness). The Center for Disease Control recommends vaccination for the flu by October 31st each year. If you are over age 65, get the high dose version of the flu vaccine or a flu vaccine that is recommended for your age group. Do not be too discouraged if you read articles that say the vaccine may not cover the flu perfectly. In my experience, even when the vaccine is not 100%, my patients who are vaccinated and get the flu have a shorter, milder course than my patients who have not been vaccinated. Also, with

Covid-19 filling our hospitals, being vaccinated for the flu can keep you out of the hospital for flu related complications.

- If you think you have the flu or any other viral infection (body aches, fever, sore throat, respiratory symptoms, nausea and/or vomiting) contact your physician as soon as possible and stay home. For the flu, certain medications can be prescribed to significantly shorten the duration of illness, but these medications must be started within the first 24-72 hours of symptoms in order to work effectively and help you recover faster.

- Wash hands or sanitize hands frequently – especially during cold and flu season. Remember virus can be found on doorknobs, desktops, and office phones among other places. Do not touch your face, eyes, nose or mouth without washing hands first if you are out in public. During the initial weeks of Covid-19, I was amazed at how often I touched my face. It is a hard habit to break, but with mindfulness you can accomplish it.

- Drink plenty of hydrating fluids. Remember, coffee, tea and soda are all mildly dehydrating. I am not suggesting you forgo them completely. In fact, tea with honey can help alleviate a sore throat. And honey has antibacterial and antiviral properties to boot. But I am recommending that you drink more water along with your tea, coffee and soda.

- Sleep with a humidifier. Viruses replicate more efficiently on dry mucus membrane. Moisturizing the air makes it harder for a virus to take hold and may reduce the duration of your illness. Also, the moist air will help you feel better. Patients of mine who have weathered Covid-19 have reported to me that hot showers and hot baths helped them feel better and breathe easier.

- While you should always check with your doctor regarding their recommendation when ill, contact your doctor if symptoms last longer than 7-10 or symptoms worsen significantly.

- Rest as much as possible (hard I know). Try to get at least 7 hours of sleep each night. Don't push yourself to do everything while fighting a virus, it will only take you longer to recover.

- Remember, antibiotics do not stop or shorten the duration of a viral illness. In fact, antibiotics have the risk of side effects and should only be prescribed when clearly indicated.

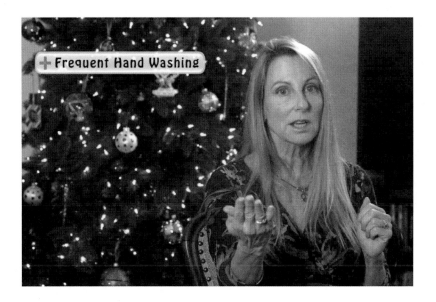

Covid 19

Now we have something more serious than the flu to worry about. And the biggest problem with this virus is that we still don't understand all there is to know about it. Health recommendations seem to change almost on a daily basis, frustrating to lay people and medical people alike. Still, we do know some things:

- Masks can decrease the risk of spreading Covid. While there are those who think otherwise, this one action is the biggest gun we currently have in our Covid-fighting arsenal. While your mask helps protect others, their mask helps protect you. Not only is mask wearing essential, but it must be worn correctly. Masks cannot do their job unless both the nose and the mouth are covered.

- Vaccines are coming, and may be a staple by the time you read this book. But again, Covid will not be the last novel virus to come along and hopefully we will have learned a lesson about personal responsibility and the loving gift we can offer by caring not only for our own health, but also for the health of others (even those we may never meet).

- Hand washing and sanitizing is essential. Remember, viruses live on surfaces like gas pumps, escalator handrails, doorknobs, anything that other hands may touch.

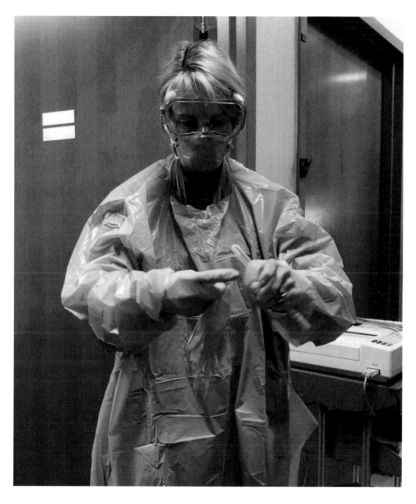

Testing For Covid 19

Healthy On The Job

Working From Home

Working from home became the norm for many employees during the Covid pandemic. My husband told me he will never go back to the office and now runs his law practice almost entirely from our living room couch. There are probably hundreds of thousands if not millions of employees who will do the same. While working from home has its benefits in saved commute times and lower dry-cleaning bills, there are some drawbacks.

- Social Isolation: Working with others gives us a camaraderie that working at home alone cannot provide. Especially for those who live alone, working with others may provide the majority of regular social interaction. For those who work at home, having outside social contact with family and friends is important. Meaningful social relationships not only boot the immune system and help maintain optimum physical health, but also play an important role in mental and spiritual wellbeing.

- Blurring of Work/Home Boundary: When we work outside the home there is a boundary between work life and home life. That boundary becomes blurred and sometimes disappears completely when working from home. Everyone needs a breather sometimes, so it is important to try and maintain a boundary. This can be done by having a cut off time or, when that is not possible, incorporating a routine that signifies the end of the workday.

- Weight Gain: Working from home means there is a refrigerator and a pantry available to you at a seconds notice. Many of my patients who now work from home notice weight gain because of this proximity. Add to that the decrease in actual movement required when working from home, and you have double trouble. Maintaining regular meal times and taking time to exercise can help stop the slide toward weight gain.

Sleep Like A Baby

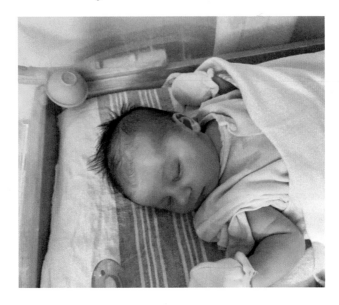

Getting a good night's sleep can be the difference between life and death, at least it almost was for me. I was driving into work at 6:15 am in the drizzling rain. My music wouldn't play properly and I was behind a very slow driver. I remember thinking *I hope this isn't foreshadowing of a bad day*, never imagining how bad it would actually get. I entered the freeway and after a few miles I was driving past an 18-wheeler when the semi stopped following the roadway and came into my lane. Without thinking or even looking, I swerved into the fast lane, but the truck kept on coming. Right before it hit my car and drove me up onto the median, I thought *I'm going to be crushed.* A moment later the 18-wheeler slammed into the side of my car and dragged it along the jersey wall about 100 yards before coming to a stop. *Oh my god, I'm still alive*, I thought. Then I saw the fire. My gas tank had ruptured and my car was burning ferociously. I had less than a minute to get out. Failure meant burning to death. I kicked the driver's side door open, but it slammed shut. I was on an angle. I kicked again, this time holding the door open with my right foot. Before I could try to throw myself up and out, I heard a voice, "Grab my arm!" he said. And I did.

I survived, but not without several fractures and some major PTSD. But what caused this near-death experience? Why did the driver come across two lanes and the shoulder without ever braking, swerving or making any attempt to avoid my car? He was sleeping. He will not drive a truck again and I have been recovering for years now, all because someone was working without getting proper rest.

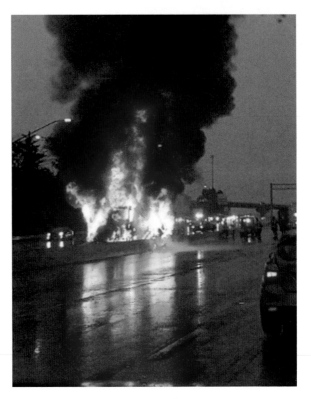

My Accident

For all of us, navigating home and work-life can be very stressful, and many people have a difficult time unwinding at night and therefore do not get a proper rest. Then there is the complication of jet lag for those employees who travel frequently for business. The following are herbal supplements than can help you get a good night's sleep and some that can help you adjust to the time changes that trigger jet lag.

- *Melatonin*: Melatonin is a hormone that our brains produce when the sun goes down. When we are young, we make a lot of it. When we get older, we make less. This may contribute to some types of sleep problems that arise with aging. To help you fall asleep faster and perhaps sleep deeper and longer, try Melatonin about 30 minutes prior to bedtime. Melatonin can help with jet lag as well if taken the first few nights after arriving from a different time zone. There is also some anecdotal evidence that is it helpful if exposed to Covid-19.

- *Chamomile Tea*: Chamomile tea can relax you prior to bedtime as well as improve your daytime performance the following day.

- *Passionflower*: Passionflower tea or a 90mg tablet at night can calm anxiety and help with sleep. It may be especially beneficial for people who cannot "turn off their mind" at night.

- *Valerian Root*: Can be taken as an oral supplement of 300 to 600 mg or you can soak 2-3 grams (2000-3000mg) of dried herbal valerian root in one cup of hot water for 10 to 15 minutes. Drink the tea or take the supplement 30 minutes to two hours before bedtime. Valerian Root also decreases anxiety quite effectively. I do warn my patients that it smells like vomit; thus taking an oral supplement, rather than the tea, may work better for those who do not like the smell of vomit (which is everyone as far as I know).

I make a sleeping concoction for my husband to take every night. He has had trouble in the past. Not falling asleep, believe me he can fall asleep during a full-blown argument, but with waking at 3 or 4 am. I give him Magnesium 400mg, Melatonin 6mg, and Valerian root 300mg (which he tolerates well as he has a diminished sense of smell). It worked pretty well, but the real cure came after he was tested for and found to have sleep apnea.

People who snore heavily or gasp for air while sleeping may think they are getting the required number of hours, but may actually have sleep apnea. If you snore loudly, have been told by a loved one that you gasp during the night, wake feeling tired, or fall asleep in the middle of an argument with your spouse, see you doctor. There are tests that can confirm sleep apnea and treatment that can help you rest more soundly.

Aromatherapy

Certain odors have been proven to trigger human responses. Because of the olfactory response (our sense of smell), some odors will help calm us down, while others increase alertness:

- *Lavender:* The smell of lavender relaxes you and can help you sleep. Putting some lavender oil on pillows or bed sheets can help you fall asleep faster and sleep deeper.

- *Peppermint:* Conversely if you did not sleep well and find yourself groggy in the morning, sniffing some peppermint can help wake you up.

Jet Lag

Many workers fly frequently for work. Jet lag can become a serious problem, interfering with memory, disturbing sleep and generally playing havoc with a person's natural circadian rhythm.

For those who fly frequently, jet lag can be avoided using a procedure that combines Melatonin and a light box (preferably blue light). This procedure requires instructions too complicated to set forth here, but the National Institute of Health site below has complete instructions regarding jet lag and its prevention. http://www.ncbi.nlm.nih.gov/pmc/articles/PMC2829880/

Healthy On The Job

Herbs To Avoid

Herbs are not necessarily benign: many are as potent as prescription drugs and some can be dangerous, even deadly. The following are herbs that were once recommended, but are now known to cause serious side effects and should be avoided.

- *Kava*: Once recommended as a sleep aid, this supplement can cause liver failure and may worsen depression. Not safe to take orally.

- *Comfry*: This herb is unsafe to take as it also can cause severe liver damage

- *Tryptophan*: OK to get naturally in food (like turkey and milk), but do not take this supplement as an oral capsule or pill as it has been linked to a disorder called EMS, a serious neurological condition with symptoms that include fatigue, intense muscle pain, nerve pain, swelling of the joints and damage to heart and liver.

- *Chaparral* – an anti-inflammatory herbal supplement that can cause severe and even fatal liver damage if take orally.

- *St Johns Wart* – helps some with depression (although severe depression should be treated by your doctor) but interacts with several other medications (including birth control pills) so if you are going to take it, discuss with your physician first.

Medication Help

Sometimes OTC sleep aids – which are mostly antihistamines – are necessary. If these also fail to work, short-term prescription medication may be indicated. Discuss this with your doctor should you feel the need for prescription medication help. Be aware though, that many prescription medications for sleep are in the class of medication called benzodiazepines or hypnotics - these medications may impact daytime performance, cause short-term memory loss, and possibly increase the risk of developing Alzheimer's disease in the future.

Sleep Hygiene

Besides using herbs, aromatherapy, and relaxation techniques to encourage better sleep, certain behaviors and strategies known as *sleep hygiene* can make a real impact on how fast you fall asleep and how long you remain sleeping:

- A warm bath before bedtime may help you relax.

- Set the bedroom thermostat at a comfortable temperature. Many people sleep better in a cooler room – try 68 degrees or cooler.

- Background white noise like a fan or a sleep machine may help you sleep better and reduce nighttime awakenings. I can't sleep without it. If you go out of town and have a smart phone, there are apps that play all night and can be a lifesaver in a noisy hotel.

- Keep the bedroom dark. Cover lights from the TV or other electronic equipment. I made felt covers for the alarm box and the Roomba vacuum robot in our bedroom.

- Avoid caffeine, nicotine and other stimulants several hours before bedtime.

- Do not use electronic devices the hour before sleeping, including reading on the kindle or iPad - there is evidence that the light from these devices can cause insomnia.

- Don't exercise too late at night – the earlier you exercise the better. Late exercise tends to stimulate and this can lead to difficulty falling asleep.

- Avoid a heavy meal or excessive snacking too close to bedtime. Also limit fluid intake in the 1-2 hours prior to bedtime to prevent nighttime awakenings due to a full bladder.

Naps

Naps can be extremely beneficial, and may even boost brainpower. The length of your nap and the type of sleep you get will help determine the brain-boosting benefits. A power nap of 10-20 minutes will allow you to awaken alert. It can also contribute to your ability to learn a motor skill like playing an instrument, typing or learning a new sport.

Longer naps help boost memory and enhance creativity. Taking a 30–60-minute nap will help with memorization and allow you to cement new learning.

A 60-to-90-minute nap benefits the brain by allowing it to form new connections and solve creative problems.

Stress Reduction

Overall, reducing stress leads to a healthier immune system, decreased rates of illness and injury, and increased psychological wellbeing. Less stressful work environments also increase employee morale. One or more of the following are good strategies to reduce stress:

- Aromatherapy can help relieve stress. Certain aromas (like lavender) have been shown to reduce stress levels.

- Listen to music and dance.

- Laughter can reduce the physical effects of stress (like fatigue) on the body

- Drink black tea, it can lower cortisol levels and promote greater feelings of relaxation

- Chewing gum can also lower cortisol

- Get a massage.

- Get or give a hug (just get permission first)

- Spend time with an animal (especially a dog)

- Keep a journal

- Take a walk (outside is best, it's good for your soul)

- Meditate

Sample Meditations

Muscle Relaxation

Lie in a comfortable position in bed or in a chair and start with the toes. Tense the muscles of the toes to the count of 10 and then relax. Feel warmth in the relaxed toes. Then tense the muscles in the feet just as you did the toes, slowly moving up your body relaxing the legs, torso, arms, shoulders, and neck until you have reached the top of your head. Then feel the warmth. Begin again in your toes and move up through the same pathway until you are warm from toes to head.

Breathing Meditation

Sit with your eyes partially or completely closed and turn your attention to your breathing. Breathe naturally, preferably through your nose, and become aware of the feeling your breath makes as it goes in and out, but do not try to control your breathing. Feeling the sensation of breathing is the object of this meditation.

The mind is very busy, and at first it may seem like it becomes even busier as you lessen outside stimulation. There is a temptation to daydream with your thoughts, but try to resist and go back to focusing on the sensation of just breathing in and out. If you realize that the mind has wandered, simply refocus on breathing. You can do this meditation for a few minutes to calm and center yourself during the day.

Guided Meditation

Some people have trouble with a breathing meditation. I am one of those people. But I have developed a kind of guided meditation that works for me; I will give you an example of it below. Of course, you are free to develop your own meditation or go online and download an audio file of a meditation that works well for you.

Take some deep breaths….in silently through your nose to the count of 5, hold your breath for 4 seconds, then breath audibly out through your mouth to the count of 6…until you have a feeling of quietness. Now as you maintain that feeling of quietness, I want you to imagine you are standing at the top of a bluff looking down to a small inlet with a beach. It is calm and peaceful and you can hear the waves breaking gently at the water's edge below. Now start walking down the path to the beach. As you walk, feel yourself becoming more and more relaxed. Feel your bare feet on the ground and the warm sand. Your path is winding and between two bluffs, but every now and then you come to a clearing and you can see the sun glimmering off the water below. As you relax further and further, you get closer and closer to the beach. When you approach the edge of the sea you notice that instead of sand, the floor beneath the water is covered in tiny crystals. Some are pink, and some are blue and some are purple. There are many colors there and each color imbues a specific power. Perhaps today you need wisdom – if so, walk into the water and feel yourself floating above the pink crystals. Feel yourself becoming wiser as the power of the crystals engulfs your body. Or perhaps you need healing. If so, go to the blue crystals and feel their power as they slowly heal you of your physical or emotional pain. As you float there and absorb the power, relax even further. Breath in and out, enjoy floating in the warm water until you feel ready to resume life.

Of course, you can make the crystals any color and give them any power you desire. Or you can make up your own guided meditation. The important thing is to find something that works for you.

Positive Visualization

Positive visualization has been shown to be a very effective strategy in accomplishing personal as well as work-place goals and even helps reduce anxiety and stress. In one study, golfers who visualized playing a round perfectly over time performed better than similar golfers who actually practiced. Visualization of your own goals and desires accomplishes some very important things:

- Presets your orientation toward success

- Starts your subconscious working on creating ideas and strategies to help you accomplish your goals (like during a nap, maybe, or before bedtime).

- Helps you visualize the steps necessary to accomplish your goals

- Helps you clarify and focus so that you have a clear idea of where you are going and what it will look like when you get there

- Opens your mind to recognize that what may appear to be random events are actually the universe sending you opportunities to make your goals and dreams a reality

- Draws people and resources into your life that can help you accomplish your goals.

- Motivates you to act

I recommend performing visualization exercises at night before sleep. I believe this gets your subconscious working all night while you sleep. I used this visualization technique at age 45 after the breakup of my marriage, while I was living in a small apartment in Los Angeles and working as a nurse practitioner. At that point I decided to go to medical school - which had been my life dream. Many people though I was delusional. Every night I imagined myself graduating from medical school and every day I took steps to make that dream a reality. I entered medical school at age 49 and graduated when I was 53. I am living proof that visualization works.

Protect Your Hearing

- The National Institute of health estimates that 15% of Americans between the ages of 20-69 (about 26 million people) have hearing loss that may be caused by exposure to noise at work or during leisure activities. But how can you know when noise is harmful?

- It helps to know how we measure sound and at what level noise can cause damage that could result in hearing loss or tinnitus (ringing or buzzing in the ear). Sound is measured in decibels – and sounds of less than 75 decibels rarely cause damage – even after long exposure. So, for instance, a pin dropping on a floor is 10 decibels, a computer humming approximately 40 decibels, normal conversation 60 decibels, the same level of noise as an air-conditioner. Noise from heavy city traffic is 85 decibels, a food processor is 95 decibels and a gunshot is 150 decibels.

- Over time, exposure to noises above the 85-decibel level can be damaging to the ear. And the decibels that you are exposed to are cumulative. The problem is that hearing loss from noise exposure is insidious and many people do not realize until hearing is very impaired.

- If you work in an environment where noise is an issue, ear protection is essential. There are several types of hearing protection, but the best hearing protector is the one that is comfortable and convenient and that you will wear every time you are in an environment with hazardous noise.

Some Types Of Ear Protection

- Expandable earplugs conform to the wearer's ear canal. There are different sized plugs so that people with smaller ear canals do not have to wear plugs that are too large and vice versa.

- Pre-molded reusable plugs are made of plastic, rubber or silicone. Because we are not completely symmetrical beings, different sized plugs may be needed for each ear as a complete seal is needed to protect hearing. Advantages of pre-molded plugs are that they are inexpensive, reusable, washable, and convenient to carry.

- Canal caps have an earplug that is attached to a headband of sorts that can be worn behind the neck or under the chin. This is convenient for people who work in intermittently noisy offices. When there is less noise, you can pull them out and let them hang around the neck until they are needed again.

- Earmuffs come in many models from large ear covers to low profile with small cups that are quite discrete. Some muffs include electronic devices to allow communication between employees. Earmuffs may not be best for men

Healthy On The Job

with beards or employees who wear glasses. For these individuals, other forms of ear protection may work better.

Protect Your Eyes

Everyone who works on a computer daily has probably rubbed their eyes at the end of the day and wondered, "What's wrong with my eyes?" Turns out, there is a medical term for what ails you: *computer vision syndrome.* The symptoms of this syndrome include dry eyes, eye pain, redness, dryness, blurring of vision and double vision. But what can you do if your job involves computer use? What can you do to protect yourself?

Have A Yearly Eye Examination

Seeing your eye doctor helps differentiate true vision problems that may require prescription glasses from computer vision syndrome. Some people need to have computer glasses in order to properly see the computer without leaning forward or straining. Computer glasses may be purchased without an eye exam, but the best pair will be one prescribed by your eye doctor.

Some computer glasses have a tint to decrease computer glare. Glare on the computer screen occurs when overhead lighting is brighter than the computer screen. This could be from overhead lighting (especially florescent lights) or from a nearby window.

48

Use of screen filters can also reduce glare and reflection of the computer screen, but should be used as a supplement to reducing glare and not a replacement for poor lighting of the room. If possible, dim the lighting in the room.

Blue Light Blocking Glasses

While there is a lack of evidence regarding blue light blocking glasses, some people swear by them (one of them is my medical assistant). If, like me, you read before bedtime on a device, blue light blocking glasses might make it easier to sleep. Studies have shown that blocking blue light before bedtime may increase the natural production of melatonin. But you should know the American Academy of Ophthalmology does not recommend these glasses and instead recommends limiting screen time. That is not always possible or desirable, so for those who cannot or will not limit screen time, they could help. Otherwise, the American Academy of Ophthalmology also recommends taking these steps:

- Use a matte screen filter on the screen to reduce glare.

- Use artificial tears when your eyes feel dry.

- Pay attention to the lighting in the room where you work. You might try increasing your screen contrast.

- If you wear contact lenses, give your eyes a break by wearing glasses now and then.

Use Good Body Mechanics

A normal computer sits about 20-26 inches from your eyes. The perfect angle at which to view the computer is such that the middle of the screen is about 5-6 inches below eye level. The U.S. Department of Labor's Occupational Safety & Health Administration (OSHA) recommends the following to use your computer safely at work:

- Sit with your head and neck upright and in-line with your torso. Do not crane your head forward or tilt back to see the screen.

- Face the computer screen directly. Avoid viewing your screen with your head turned or your back twisted.

- Keep your elbows comfortably close to your body.

- Have a chair that provides good support for your lower back and has a cushioned seat with a contoured front edge.

- Keep the mouse close to your keyboard so you don't have to reach for it.

- Position your computer display so the top of the screen is at or slightly below eye level.

- Adjust the position of your display to prevent reflections of overhead and outdoor lighting appearing on your screen.

- Put your monitor close enough to your eyes so you can comfortably read text on the screen without leaning forward.

- When working with print documents, use a document holder that positions them at the same height and distance as your computer screen.

- Use a hands-free headset when talking on the phone while working at your computer.

Other suggestion to avoid repetitive action injury include:

- Tap computer keys softly and do not squeeze the mouse (hard for those of us who learned to type on a typewriter)

- Move smoothly and do not jerk while performing tasks.

- A cold environment stiffens muscles and can cause workplace injuries. If possible keep office temperature comfortable. If not possible, keep hands and fingers warm with gloves

Healthy On The Job

- If you are exposed to vibration try to take breaks to limit continuous exposure.

- Break up repetitious work. Take a break from looking at the computer every 20 minutes or so and look around to exercise eye muscles

- Relax muscles as much as possible. Don't constantly tense muscles, but instead keep limbs and shoulders relaxed.

- Keep wrists, elbows and shoulders in a neutral position – do not keep joints in awkward or uncomfortable position for long periods of time.

- For wrists and elbows especially, limit contact with hard or sharp surfaces.

Body Mechanics For Lifting

According to OSHA, lost work due to back injury or other work-related musculoskeletal injuries cost businesses over 18 billion dollars a year, more than twice that when taking production losses into account. But as a physician who treats patients for back pain and other musculoskeletal injuries, the cost to business is only the tip of the iceberg. Pain and suffering from one wrong move can devastate a person's quality of life.

Before becoming a physician, I was a hospital nurse and as such I took many body mechanics courses. Had I known then what I know now, I would have been much more careful during my working life. The following are suggestions to follow to help prevent injury at work through good body mechanics, good decision-making, and simple treatments for minor strains or sprains.

When lifting, scope out the area where you are moving the object and make sure you have a clear, unobstructed path. Shoes should be non-slip and feet should be about shoulder length apart, with one foot slightly more forward. Move yourself close to the object. If the object is on a table or other elevated structure move it against your body before lifting. If it is on the floor, make sure you use your legs and core (abdominal muscles) to lift. Do not stoop over with legs straight, but bend legs and use them to help you lift the object. Make sure you have a good grip before attempting to lift the object. Do not strain. If it is too heavy find someone to help you or use a moving device. Even a rolling office chair can be used if that is all you have.

When carrying something do not twist or bend from the back. Move your feet if you have to place something to one side or the other. Twisting while lifting is a recipe for back pain disaster. Despite following all these steps, you could experience bouts of mild to moderate back pain, even if your job is not terribly physical. I recommend that my patients ice the back for 10-15 minutes immediately if they feel like they have strained their back muscles and repeat icing again at home when they have finished the workday. If no contraindications to medication, I also have them take a NSAID like Ibuprofen 600mg to decrease inflammation. Sleep position at night can help or hurt as well. Sleeping on a firmer mattress on your back or on your side are preferable sleep positions for back health. Side sleepers should put a pillow between their legs. Stomach sleeping and/or using a large pillow can aggravate back pain.

When To See A Doctor About Back Pain

If you have severe pain, pain from your back that radiates

54

down your leg, numbness or weakness in the leg, loss of bladder or bowel control, or pain getting worse or persisting for more than a few weeks, see your doctor. Certainly, if symptoms are not this severe, but you are concerned, contact your doctor for further instruction.

Mindfulness And Safety In The Workplace

There are many accident prevention guidelines, pamphlets and recommendations to decrease accidents at work that are beyond the scope of this book. However, I do want to stress that many, if not most accidents and injuries on the job could be prevented with mindfulness.

One day, long before my accident, I drove from my house early in the morning to work. I was thinking about my coming day and realized when I arrived at work that I was completely unaware of driving to work. I did not remember one turn, one stop light…it was as if I was at home one minute and transported magically to work the next. Often when we are preoccupied or doing repetitive tasks with which we are very familiar, we go on autopilot. This is a recipe for accident disaster.

The definition I like for mindfulness in the context of accident prevention is paying attention in a particular way: on purpose, in the present moment, without judgment. For employees to be

55

mindful at work requires a personal commitment to stay in the present moment, stay focused, and be keenly aware of the work environment. Strategies that stress healthy behaviors both physical and psychological, boost stamina, and allow for recharging and relaxation motivate employees to stay mindful. But it is not just the individual employee who must remain mindful: the organization itself must set the example by adopting a policy of mindfulness. To promote organizational mindfulness employers should:

- Encourage reporting of problems

- Commit to safety

- Have realistic and flexible processes to deal with risk

- Improve practices when risk is identified

All of us allow our minds to drift at times, and studies show that a "breather" every so often helps boost productivity. But many accidents at work happen even when organizational accident prevention programs are in place and being followed. Mindfulness training in the workplace from the top of the organization down could potentially eliminate many work place accidents.

Gun Violence At Work

Unfortunately, we live in a time and a place where workplace shootings are a reality. Over the past several years there have been several multiple death shootings in the workplace in which hundreds of people were killed, some employees and some customers. An FBI study of all shootings between 2000 and 2013 showed the majority of incidents—45.6% of the 160—occurred in an environment related to commerce. The second most common incident locations were in educational environments (24.4%).

Multiple shootings at concerts and church have also been reported in the news. Slowly there has begun to be a paradigm shift in how one should react to gunman at work or school. This is much like the paradigm shift that happened after the skyjacking of 9/11. Prior to these passengers on a plane would cooperate in the hopes that they would be safe once the plane landed. When hijacked airplanes were used as weapons, flying into buildings, everything changed. Now, I do not believe passengers would sit by and allow a plane to be hijacked without a fight.

There have been many deadly mass shootings both in workplaces and in schools. One deadly college shooting in Oregon where many students and faculty were killed exemplifies why this shift is evolving. A gunman, after entering the school and shooting a teacher in the head, ordered the rest of the class to get on the ground. After they got down, he instructed those who were Christians to stand up. He then shot them one-by-one, even stopping to reload.

One student, who hid in a different classroom, told authorities that when she and her classmates heard the shooting, they dropped to the floor and huddled behind backpacks and desks. Could any of them have done something different to save their lives? Possibly yes.

The analysis of what happened in Oregon can identify strategies that workplace employees can incorporate to protect themselves and others. The first advice when confronted with a situation like the one described above is to stay calm, or at least as calm as possible. Staying calm allows you to think - of a way out, of a potential escape, of a weakness the gunman might have and how you could exploit that weakness to your own advantage – anything that might give you an opportunity to stay safe and alive.

Second, the normal inclination of a group of people confronted by a gunman is to huddle together. Ironically that instinct to stay close to others is the worst thing you could do. Huddling together gives the gunman an easy target and keeps you all in the kill zone. Drifting apart or moving away from others

Healthy On The Job

actually makes it more difficult for the gunman to hit multiple people.

Third, as a last resort, when there is an active shooter in the building actually shooting and killing people, it is better to fight for your life than passively wait to die. For years we have told people to lock down and hide. Hiding behind a desk or a backpack will offer little protection if a shooter intent on killing enters your building. The gunman in the Oregon shooting stopped to reload several times. It is possible that he could have been stopped had he been rushed during these reloading intervals. Many reputable agencies, including homeland security, recommend that first and foremost, try to escape the area. If you are in an area far from the shooter, get out, even if others will not come with you. Leave your valuables and cell phones behind if you have to. Help others who might need your help to get away as well.

If you are unable to escape and in a visible area like a hallway, try to get to a room where you can hide. Lock and/or barricade the door and silence your cell phone. The last thing you need is your phone ringing as the gunman looks for victims. Remain quiet, but be prepared to fight if the shooter enters the room.

If there are several people in the room, make a plan. Place the stronger individuals off to the side of the entry doorway in a

Healthy On The Job

position to surprise and take down the shooter should he enter. This is also in line with the instructions of Homeland Security:

- When the shooter is at close range and you cannot flee, your chance of survival is much greater if you try to incapacitate him/her.

- If you can flee, running from the shooter in a zig-zag manner may be your best option. Statistically a shooter has less chance of wounding or killing you if you run away in this manner. If you cannot flee and the shooter is intent on killing, do whatever you can to incapacitate the gunman.

- If possible, your work should have a plan and some education in place regarding an active shooter on the premises. For instance, a grocery store could have a code that when announced over the intercom would warm employees that there is a shooter in the building. I will admit though that the more than 40+ years I have worked in medicine, only once was I offered education by my workplace about what to do if a gunman enters the workplace. So, like those of you in similar circumstances, I advise you to make your own plan. I have a plan with my medical assistant – she and I along with any patients will head to my office if there is even a hint that someone is in

60

our building with a gun. We work in what used to be a Giant Supermarket with multiple hallways and individual pods with exam rooms and physician offices. There are probably more than 40 doctors in our building. It would be very difficult if not impossible to for us to leave the building safely. Once in my office, we will barricade the door and call for help.

I have been in a situation early in my career when a gun wielding man came to our clinic. It was a gang issue when I worked in Los Angeles. One gang member was there with his wife and another from a different gang came with his wife and there was an altercation in the waiting room. One couple left, but the man returned with a gun. Fortunately, no one was hurt and we were all advised to go home by the police. Today a situation like that would likely end in tragedy.

Working Alone

Sometimes when working late or arriving early to work, one might be alone when entering or leaving the office. Some work sites have security on site. Still, there are a few safety precautions to note here:

- Be aware of your surroundings. Too often, we are looking at our cell phones, texting or planning the day's agenda in our mind. You must stay aware of your surroundings to protect yourself. Make eye contact with those around you. Many times, an attacker will avoid a victim who appears confident or who has been looking at them directly.

- Listen to your intuition. My ex-husband, a police officer, told me that victims of crime often told him that they had an intuition or felt uncomfortable but did not act on their feelings. For instance, one woman was waiting for an elevator and when it opened, she felt uncomfortable, but worried how it might appear if she did not get in. She was attacked in that elevator. Her intuition was right, but she ignored it. If you find yourself feeling uncomfortable, listen to your intuition. It could save your life. If you are walking to your car and you think that someone walking nearby might try to hurt you: get to your car, get in and lock the door. It doesn't matter if you think you look silly or rude. What matters is staying safe.

- Many experts, including my ex-husband, also advised the following: If someone attempts to abduct you, never leave the site of abduction even if the attacker has a knife or a gun. Victims who allow an attacker to remove them from the original crime scene are 10 times more likely to be injured or killed. Better to be shot or stabbed in the parking lot of a public building than taken to a remote area.

- If you are able, run! Experts say than an assailant with a gun will only hit you 4 out of 100 times if you run. Escape the area if possible.

- If you are unable to run and you think you have a chance to get away by fighting: Fight. Many experts recommend self-defense courses for women, but frankly most men would benefit as well. These courses should prepare you to defend yourself in close quarters. If you do fight, aim for your assailant's vulnerable areas: eyes, head (nose especially), groin and the instep of the foot.

- If your car does not unlock automatically, carry your car keys in your hand when you go to the car. This prevents fumbling to find the keys if you need to get into your car fast.

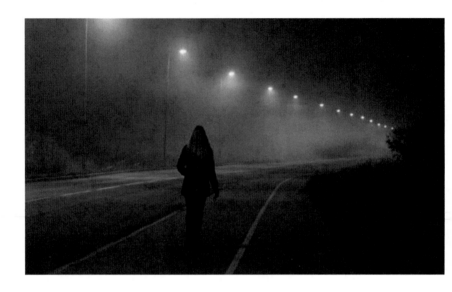

Boost Brain Power

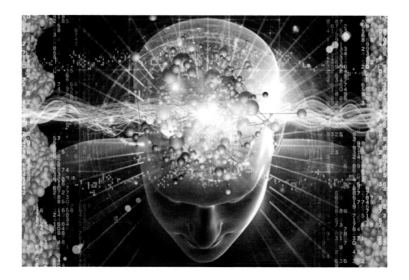

Keeping your brain healthy improves overall health. To do so, requires certain dietary and lifestyle commitments: Be mindful of what you eat - diets high in salt, saturated fats and sugar actually **shrink** the brain over time. To grow the brain instead:

- Get enough DHA Omega 3 – eat two servings of fish a week and take 1000mg of DHA daily (more if you can't commit to eating the fish)

- Fill up on Flavonoids - green tea, quercetin (found in apple skins), beets, blueberries, caffeine (about 200mg daily – the amount in one cup of coffee) cocoa, pecans, red grapes, spinach, and tomatoes all improve blood flow to the brain.

- Don't skip the important vitamins your brain needs:
    - B12
    - Vitamin D
- Drink in moderation: Moderate alcohol intake is believed to protect brain and nervous system function
- Meditate to help grow your brain
- Grow your brain with Tai Chi, Yoga and Mindfulness
- Use positive visualization and gratitude
- Engage emotionally with others
- Perform memory exercises
- Decrease stress and treat Depression - both over time will shrink your brain

When I started medical school, I was 49 years old and worried that I would never keep up with my classmates who were 25 years younger. How could I stay competitive? I ended up doing some research and purchased a supplement called phosphatidyl serine 300mg. This was supposed to help me with age related memory loss and make me sharper.

About two months into school, I could feel myself making

connections faster and also remembering better, but at the time I didn't think it was the supplement, I thought I had opened a door to learning in my brain. A few months later I ran out of the supplement and had no time to get it refilled. I felt myself getting slower (like the sad climax of *Flowers for Algernon*). At the time I thought, *what's wrong with me? Maybe at my age I only have six good months and I've run out of steam.*

Finally, when we had a break, I bought more phosphatidyl serene and started taking it again. In two weeks, I felt that sharp feeling coming back and I thought, *it's the phosphatidyl serine.* I have been taking it ever since. I make my husband take it too (sense a pattern here?)

Unexpected Problems

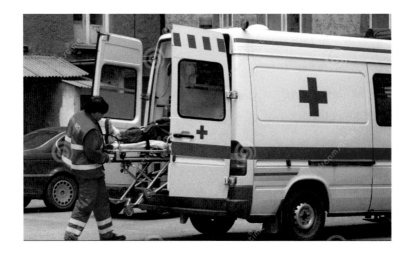

Unexpected problems can always arise at the workplace. It helps to have a primary care physician who you know to treat emergencies and help navigate the medical system when specialized care is necessary. Some, if not everyone in the work system, should know CPR and be able to provide it in an emergency. If training everyone is a hardship, then a few people in each area should be trained. An AED (automatic external defibrillator) should be available on every floor as well as some basic first aid supplies. Everyone should know how to access life-saving equipment.

Healthy On The Job

The intention of this book has been to give you strategies to stay healthy in your life, both at work and at home. Taken together, the diet, lifestyle, immune boosting and stress reducing techniques outlined in these pages can significantly improve the health of both the individual and the organization. By preventing illness, productivity is enhanced and sick time is limited, substantially benefiting everyone.

Healthy On The Job

Made in the USA
Monee, IL
16 July 2021